Reset

Omar Al-Duri

PASSIONPRENEUR
P U B L I S H I N G

Reset
Copyright © 2018 Omar Al-Duri
First published in 2019

ISBN
Paperback: 978-0-6485050-7-5
E-book: 978-0-6485050-8-2

Because of the dynamic nature of the Internet, any web addresses or links contained in this book may have changed since publication and may no longer be valid. The information in this book is based on the author's experiences and opinions. The views expressed in this book are solely those of the author and do not necessarily reflect the views of the publisher; the publisher hereby disclaims any responsibility for them.

The author of this book does not dispense any form of medical, legal, financial, or technical advice either directly or indirectly. The intent of the author is solely to provide information of a general nature to help you in your quest for personal development and growth. In the event you use any of the information in this book, the author and the publisher assume no responsibility for your actions. If any form of expert assistance is required, the services of a competent professional should be sought.

Publishing information
Publishing, design, and production facilitated by Passionpreneur Publishing
www.PassionpreneurPublishing.com

Melbourne, VIC I Australia

Dedication

*I dedicate this book to my mother
Fatemah and wife Maria.
Paradise lies under the feet of a mother.
To the world, you are a mother. To a
family, you are the world.
Maria, you are my best friend and
knowing you are present and willing to
lift me up when I'm feeling down let's
me know I'm not alone and fills my heart
with gratitude and love.
Thank you both for redefining the true
meaning of unconditional love and
allowing me to feel alive.*

Ironically, that was one of the best things that could have happened as it taught me to empathize with those who don't always have the answer and approach them with a sense of understanding and care. The more I listened, the more disciplined I became on how to face an issue or problem. Apart from school and university, a lot of life lessons were self-taught through trial and error. I have always believed that timing is everything. As a result, I left home and moved to a completely foreign culture in order to pursue a dream of opening one of the first holistic training facilities in the Middle East.

Throughout my time in working in various roles and facilities in Europe and the United Arab Emirates (UAE), I was able to understand the industry on a global level and identify that the UAE was evolving at a rapid speed and needed to focus more on well-being, followed by bespoke functional training. Over a decade ago, I created a concept in the heart of Dubai—Platform 3, also known as P3, a first of its kind, based on three essential platforms:

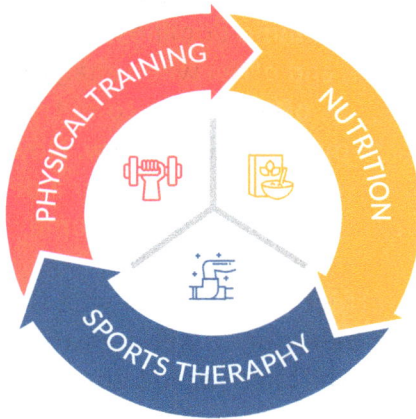

After only two months of being fully operational, I was recognized by Shape Middle East as Personal Trainer of the Year—2011. Shortly after the award, P3 had been nominated as one of the top five facilities within the region for high-end functional fitness. Amid the highs of creating a business in a cut-throat industry, five years later, I hit a low after losing my business, which resulted in my falling out of love with the industry. However, like William F. O'Brien once mentioned, "Better to try and fail than fail to try." The experience of failing to manage my own facility taught me where my passion truly lies within the fitness industry, and that is focusing on an individual's well-being and development, rather than the business-management element.

As you read through the different chapters, keep in mind the concept behind dominos. The domino effect is common in life, and often when analyzing a program or daily habits, we often revert to nutrition and how you fuel your body to tackle the day. Now I'm no doctor, but I have been a patient for over a decade, which I now see as being a student of the game.

The domino effect states that when you make a change to one behavior, it will activate a chain reaction and cause a shift in related behaviors as well. You may have heard similar comparisons to "the snowball effect" or "chain reactions." The methodology behind using dominos throughout this book is to symbolize each pillar's individual importance and the magnitude of the chain as a holistic approach. If one isn't mastered, it tends to set us back, which is why I will do my best to simplify them and explain how they complement one another.

The analogy of dominos can apply to many factors when putting in perspective. For example, meditating and giving myself personal time to balance myself in the morning results in setting the tone for the rest of the day, enabling me to be more productive and in a better state of mind. Now in order to do so, I would have to give myself more time to channel that. Whereas if I were to miss my alarm, I may start to get agitated by the fact that I am running late, get stuck in traffic, and probably react in an unnecessary manner to a colleague or person passing by at that moment. So, enabling myself that time to focus on that domino helps me manage things better in order to smash the day ahead!

This book will look to explore the different elements of one's journey toward well-being through five different dominos. Explored throughout those dominos will be the highs, the lows, the mental and physical challenges, the diets, the myths, and, most importantly, how to habitually RESET your environment.

Domino 1—70/30 Rule

70 percent of abs are made in the kitchen versus 30 percent bullshit.

—Omar Al-Duri

Introduction

After your formal education, you enter the most critical phase in your life—a second, practical education known as the apprenticeship. The dangers are many. If you are not careful, you will succumb to insecurities and become embroiled in emotional issues and conflicts that will dominate your thoughts; you will develop fears and learning disabilities that you will carry with you throughout your life. Before it is too late, you must learn the lessons and follow the path established by the greatest masters, past and present, a kind of ideal apprenticeship that transcends all fields.

—Robert Greene from *The Concise Mastery*

The obsession of being the perfect guardian, father figure, or coach comes through the fact that I didn't have the privilege of having my father around throughout my childhood.

Domino 1
Our Body Will Always Reflect What We Consistently Do

ONE OF LIFE'S challenges, since we are born, is striking a balance when brought into this world. It starts with the responsibility our parents have when bringing us into this world and feeding us. Some of the readers reading this will understand that the sense of accountability quadruples if you thought it was tough managing your own nutrition. The parents play the role of coaches in our early years, rewarding us with something "yummy" if we are good, right? I got rewarded with a lot of food—so much that I was that kid!

Now, by no means do I regret any part of my childhood because it was part of my growing up and learning! However, I can now identify patterns from my childhood that can impede longevity. Eating was a hobby, and emotional eating was the effect I encountered when things didn't go as planned. How do we pick up these habits? Could a parent or younger version of me relate to this?

It's only when I entered my teen years and had to do my weigh-in before making that jump to high school from primary school did I dread the day we had to record all our metrics in public. Facing that was probably a wakeup call, when I heard the number 67 kg in front of all the students and teachers. Alongside this, I was too big to play the sport we all loved and grew up to—football! Yes, I played in goal because I figured that even if I couldn't match the other players physically or technically, I could use my weight and size to cover most of the goal and be a goalkeeper. Whether it was lack of knowledge or experience, I soon began my journey toward understanding more about refueling the body and what was required to strike the right balance. Having been a human guinea pig throughout my life, I chose to learn more about nutrition by furthering my education at university, as the more I read, the more the opinions confused me. Diets such as keto and vegan, and methods such as intermittent fasting, counting macros, and juicing were all things I tried. The knowledge of nutrition can change lives and prevent chronic diseases like heart disease and cancer, which can be later passed on to generations in the family tree. Arguably the most important chapter in the book, I tend to shy away from overusing the word diet because I feel, especially in the culture I grew up in, it has a short-term connotation when describing it. In the Middle East, it may be seen differently as compared to Europe, Africa, or America. "What's wrong? Are you ok?" Yes, I'm on a diet so can't have that.

Diet: The kind of food that a person, animal, or community habitually eats (Webster's Dictionary).

This chapter is dedicated to those who are mastering the balanced technique of nutrition. When I read into the definition of diet, the word *habitual* screams at me. Those who master nutrition strike the right balance, which isn't restricting but appears sustainable long term, promoting the term *habit*.

I have come across studies that will help you create your own positive healthy habits. Before the day and age of additives, preservatives, MSG, and the misconception of food labels, our ancestors have proven that one can be healthy.

Food for thought: Ever wondered how fresh can food be if it has a long shelf life? What chemicals are merged together to keep it alive? I will highlight the foundational principle in nutrition and how it can play a pivotal role in energy levels and in productivity at work, and how it fuels your body and helps with recovery.

"You cannot outtrain a bad diet." I trained like an animal and then fueled the incorrect way, which resulted in not being able to operate and function at optimal levels. Once I mastered that balance in being more organized and planning my fuel, the body was able to perform at such a better level, resulting in better rest. This didn't just apply to me in my athletic young days, but more as I got older. I started to realize I wasn't getting away with certain foods when digesting them. My body was responding to gluten and lactose differently, which never was the case earlier. What was wrong with me? Nothing, life!

What am I doing different now to last month or year? Let's break it down.

Calorie: A Calorie is a measure of energy (Webster's Dictionary).

The body needs a certain amount of energy to maintain its basic functions. Breathing, thinking, and even sleeping require energy.

The beauty of being able to personalize your own lifestyle is that you are in charge. The body requires a certain amount of energy to maintain its basic systems. It's harder to give an identical program to someone who lives a sedentary lifestyle than to an athlete. The reason being that their human organs and functions don't match or operate at the same levels. One would argue that nutrition is at the top of the chain in resetting your health and fitness goals. That never changes, and 70 percent of the time it is a fact! The remaining 30 percent is a combination of many factors including the BULL$#%! You read about getting a six pack in six days!

Whether it's visualizing how great you will look in your swimsuit, perform in your favorite sport, or just out-run your 3-year-old baby around the house without cutting the game short due to feeling out of breath; you cannot put a price on health and well-being.

The problem in modern society is the "fast food industry," because everyone wants results instantly without sacrificing or working for it. This prevents us from enjoying the process and passing over the knowledge and experience we learn from achieving our goals.

There is no correct or incorrect answer when planning nutritional strategies because every body type is different. Whether you choose to eliminate dairy (lactose intolerant) or meat (vegetarian) or go keto (fat diet) or count your macros (IIFYM), my advice when doing so is to strip it back bit by bit rather than going extreme and not sustaining it. The method is to allow the body to clear whatever your gut has accumulated over a period of time, which will help identify what works best for you. This enables the body to react, resulting in some drastic changes in how you look and feel without going extreme. How many years have we unconsciously fed our bodies the wrong thing? You can't expect to rectify that in a week; it takes time and discipline to be able to make positive changes.

Below you will find a number of options simplifying many of these celebrity-familiar diets currently taking over the world:

VEGAN DIET

GREENS: BROCCOLI, CUCUMBER, BRUSSEL SPROUTS, ASPARAGUS, KALE

LEGUMES: LENTILS, RED BEANS, BLACK BEANS, CHICKPEA

CALCIUM: ROCCA LEAVE, TOFU, SOY MILK, KALE, MUSTARD LEAVES

WHOLE GRAIN: BROWN RICE, FLOUR BREAD, BLACK RICE, PASTAS,SQUASH, GINGER TOMATO

COLOFUL REGGIES: RED CABBAGE, MIXED BELL PEPPERS,MIXED CARROTS

FRUITS: BANANA,STRAUBERRY,KIWI,ORANGE, POMEGRANATE, GUAVA, MELON

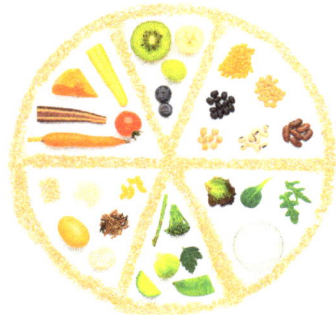

KETO DIET

PROTEIN:20%
FAT:70%
CARBS:10%

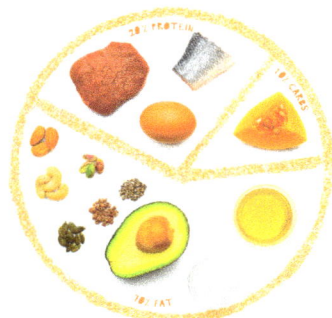

ECTOMORPH DIET

CARBS:55%

PROTEIN: 25%

FAT: 20%

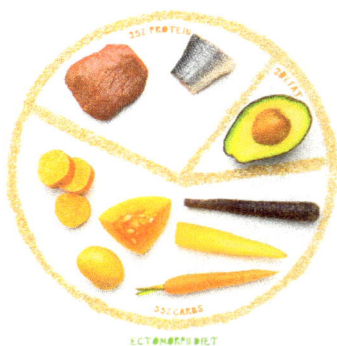

ECTOMORPH DIET

ENDOMORPH DIET

CARBS: 25%

PROTEIN: 35%

FAT: 40%

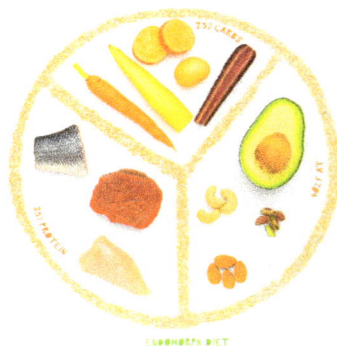

ENDOMORPH DIET

MESOMORPH DIET

CARBS: 40%
PROTEIN: 30%
FAT: 30%

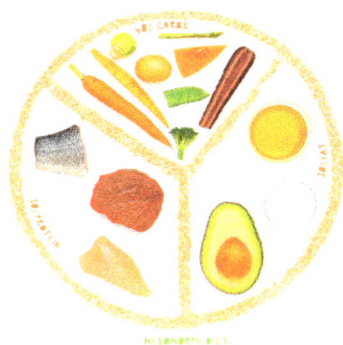

PALEO DIET

CARBS: 30%
PROTEIN: 30%
FAT: 40%

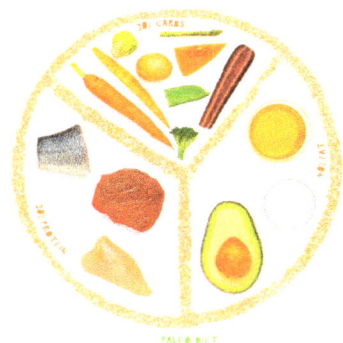

Structure Your Nutrition with Your Lifestyle

How many hours are you sitting at a desk, in the car, or on the couch? How active is your lifestyle? Do you require more calories due to the energy you need from physical activity? If getting leaner or reducing body fat specifically is your goal, how hard is it to reduce your calorie intake by 500 kcal because you had to stay late for work or missed training that day? Arnold Schwarzenegger once said,

> *Everybody has a problem with time. The day has 24 hours—we sleep 6 hours. Some may say I need 8! I say sleep a little faster. If we have 24 hours and you sleep 8 of those you have 16 hours to do your work, be with your family, learn something new which could be a new language, read a new book or even a new activity or commit to reshaping your body or living healthy. I'm going to take an hour of my day to train. It definitely is a challenge but totally doable. Hours are too precious, don't give me I have difficulty with times can't find the time— You make time!*

In the same interview, he discussed balancing his school, jobs, acting classes, and training all in the same period, which was quite inspiring and definitely helps me when I'm feeling lazy and take time for granted. While many focus on fat loss or getting leaner, one cannot ignore muscle maintenance and its effect on our everyday function. I strongly believe in getting the right balance with weight training or anaerobic training. Anaerobic exercise is a physical exercise intense enough to cause lactate to form. It is used by athletes in non-endurance sports to promote strength, speed, and power, and by bodybuilders to build muscle mass (Medical Dictionary).

Aerobic exercise is the type of moderate-intensity physical activity that you can sustain for more than just a few minutes with the objective of improving your cardiorespiratory fitness and your health (Medical Dictionary).

The food you eat determines how well you can keep a level of body fat while still feeding the muscles. The human body naturally likes to be in a state of homeostasis (remaining stable) and prefers to maintain a balance of energy (calories) in and calories out. If I have 10 kg of excess body fat to lose, I am likely to experience rapid success shedding the first 4–6 kg with the right nutrition and training. However, my body will start to recognize this and eventually go into defense mode—some refer to this as plateauing. At that stage, when restricting calories to below what the body is used to, the body adapts to conserve fuel being burned (energy out). It takes energy from muscle tissue, preserving body fat to keep vital organs warm and slowing down metabolism. So, the moral of the story is, decreasing your calories too low in the hope of burning fat may be detrimental that eventually could lead to weight gain, anxiety, or even yoyo fluctuation.

CARBS: 4 CALORIES
PROTEIN: 4 CALORIES
FAT: 9 CALORIES

All three macronutrients supply energy, with carbohydrates and protein yielding 4 calories per gram while fat yields 9 calories per gram. Each gram of protein, carbohydrate, and fat has different caloric values. Bioavailability is the body's ability to access those calories. While fat and carbs provide more energy, protein provides the structural components necessary for growth and repair of muscle tissue that is extremely important to both fat loss and muscle growth.

In this context, it's clear to see that fat provides more energy than either protein or carbohydrates. I like to call fat *the gram for gram champion* of macronutrients. The reason being that a gram of fat yields more than twice the energy of the other macros, with 97 percent being made available as energy.

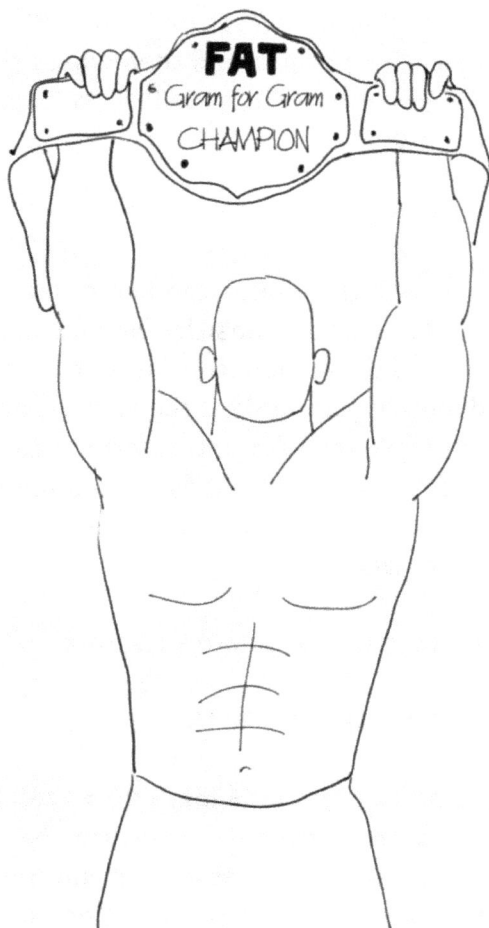

Protein and carbohydrates only have a thermogenic rating of 80 percent and 90 percent, respectively. The thermic effect of food is the energy used in digestion, absorption, and distribution of nutrients. For example, if proteins' thermic effect of food is 80 percent and I consume 100 g of protein, then where does the remaining 20 percent go? It gets lost as heat during the digestion process.

Basal Metabolism

What if having a better understanding of metabolism helped regulate a stable, healthy weight, leaving us feeling energized throughout the day with control over fat loss and muscle gain? BMR is the amount of energy your body requires each day in the form of calories to function properly while your body is at complete rest. Now with a more healthy and active lifestyle, you can burn even more while resting.

Here's a little formula for you to kick-start.

Body weight (in lbs) x 10 = BMR

EXAMPLE: Body weight (176 lbs) x 10 = 1760 (BMR)
Let's take things in perspective—nutrition has no religion, and what I mean by that is that you don't have to religiously stick to one type of nutrition plan. There are formulas such as intermittent fasting, 80/20 high

carb and low sugar diet, or a specific focus on high-fat eating. The idea is to try and test what works for your body type best. Clean eating is something many struggle to do because of many factors. How expensive is it compared to a fast-food burger? How often do you need to go to the grocery store to get fresh products?

We get bored of the same food, so go and get creative! If you're not a magician in the kitchen like me, take your partner and go to a cooking class. Enjoy the experience, and you might actually appreciate how blessed we are to have had family/friends cook for us in the past. It comes down to discipline and dedication. Make time to make it a habit to fuel the right way. Preparing your own meals and putting the time in actually does hold a high regard for accountability, which helps develop our mind-set on appreciating food more. You then develop a more efficient approach that results in productivity and time management, building a very positive habit. We all want to feel good, and our bodies deserve to function the best way possible by making subtle changes.

Gut Health: The Second Brain
How important is it to have a healthy gut? It's not just something that reduces diseases when you get it right—it really does come down to the quality of life and becoming a happier person. Since 80 percent of your immune system is located in your gut, and the digestive system is the second largest part of your neurological system,

the value and importance of the second brain is not surprising. I always say that feeling better is a lot more effective than looking better when beginning your journey of longevity in health. How many of us have reached our goals, but when reflecting on the process afterward realized how miserable we were? That really does boil down to how we feel internally rather than externally. I struggled with maintaining weight because I was a fitness ambassador before social media blew up in 2008 and reduced my weight to 75 kg, which in my mother's eyes was too skinny, bless her heart. Having been in that cycle, I didn't know any better; that resulted in many complications medically, which took a toll on my body.

Our gut is connected to every part of our body. The expression "I have a bad feeling in my gut" indicates it's a world of its own. Hence, the title "second brain" means it has a mind of its own in our gut. When we get sad and we overeat or under-eat, it's because the amount of work being done in there is phenomenal. Most of the gut flora is in your colon or your large intestine, which is the last part of the digestive process. When I think of how much is stored there when foods that are processed or unhealthy enter it makes me feel like I need something to counter that. I don't eat badly, but from time to time I do indulge and eat in moderation something that I want.

Probiotics are often overlooked when considering having a healthy gut; unfortunately, in modern society we wait until it's too late to consider them. Probiotics are live bacteria that are good for your digestive system and fight the bad bacteria in the body. Inflammation in the gut caused by a poor diet may cause allergies or leaking of the gut that can irritate the skin and cause illness. It's really worth visiting a specialist to find out which probiotic suits your body type and learning more about its benefits and, more importantly, what it can do for you in the long term.

Some of the best foods for gut health:

Fiber: Whole grains, beans, and legumes
Whole fruits and vegetables
Plant-based greens
Fermented foods: Sauerkraut, kimchi, tempeh, miso, and pickles.

My personal pick from the bunch is:

Kombucha
The fermentation process of Kombucha means the drink is rich in probiotics (living healthy bacteria) and comes along with several health benefits extending to your heart, your brain, and especially your gut. Among these benefits are liver health, type 2 diabetes, weight management, and an increase in metabolism. For optimal digestive benefits, kombucha is often consumed on an empty stomach to enable the

living healthy bacteria to reach the large intestine more easily.

Originating in the Far East over 2,000 years ago, I am not surprised at the benefits and mind-set behind the culture when viewing state of mind, metabolic rate, and overall well-being. Chef Victor Urbina who is an international chef and recognized figure in the food and beverage world creates his own, highlighting the incredible feedback he gets from his clients.

> The benefits are fantastic especially when being creative—from pineapple Kamboocha to strawberry I create it with a twist and my clients love it—seeing incredible results.

Superfoods: Increase Energy

Superfoods are extremely important when promoting daily habits because they help increase energy levels, prevent diseases such as cancer, and reduce the risk of heart disease. Antioxidants found in many superfoods may help reduce your risk of certain chronic health conditions while providing multiple health benefits. Among their many health benefits are that they pro-tect your organs from toxins, help lower cholesterol, regulate metabolism, and reduce inflammation. These powerhouses provide large quantities of antioxidants, phytochemicals (chemicals in plants responsible for colors and smells), vitamins, and minerals.

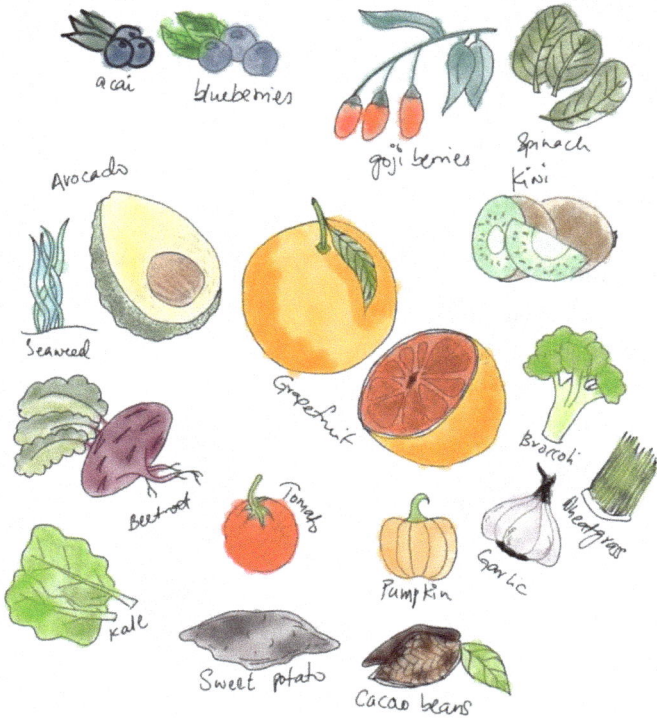

acai

blueberries

goji berries

Spinach

Avocado

Kiwi

Seaweed

Grapefruit

Broccoli

Beetroot

Tomato

Wheatgrass

Kale

Pumpkin

Garlic

Sweet potato

Cacao beans

Superfoods
Acai berries
Avocados
Blueberries
Goji berries
Kiwi
Grapefruit

Beets
Broccoli
Kale
Pumpkin
Sweet potato
Seaweed
Spinach
Tomatoes
Wheatgrass

Garlic
Cacao
Chia seed
Cinnamon
Coconut
Flaxseed
Ginger
Hemp seed
Quinoa
Turmeric

Beans
Free-range organic eggs
Greek yogurt
Green tea
Lentils
Wild fish salmon, cod, mackerel

Foods That Could Cause Fatigue and Drain Energy

White Bread
Pasta
Fried Foods
Cereals
Processed foods
White rice
Sugary foods
Cakes
Muffins
Cookies
Alcohol
High fructose corn syrup
MSG
High sodium food
Aspartame

Risk Factors

1. Going away from basics
2. Increased screen time on your phone or computer

3. Dehydration
4. Relying on sauces with high fructose corn syrup or chemicals rather than spices and herbs
5. Not having a plan and jumping ahead of the queue
6. Expecting sudden results without actually allowing the time to do so
7. Permanent assumption on a temporary emotion
8. Working so hard to increase your current standard of living that you forget to increase the standard of your well-being

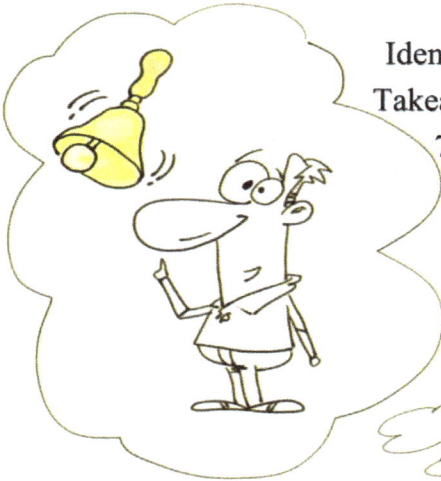

Identify Your Key
Takeaways from the
70/30 Rule

❖ Takeaway 1

❖ Takeaway 2

❖ Takeaway 3

❖ Takeaway 4

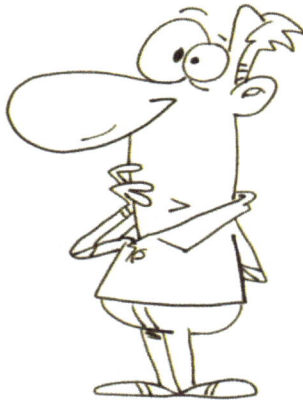

DOMINO 2: Unwind Your Mind

Mental illness is not contagious, you can't catch it by being kind.

—Unknown

Domino 2:
Mind-set—The Toughest Battle Is Your Own

AMONG THE TOUGHEST challenges I faced was the battle with my mind. The "silent killer," otherwise known as mental health, is often overseen and overlooked in modern society. Depression, losing my business, valuable close people passing away, weight gain, and a life-threatening car accident raised a lot of questions on whether life was worth living. These are issues that many people face daily, bearing stress, anxiety, and emotions on their shoulders. Not all wounds are visible, with some experiencing trauma resulting in silence, which can be challenging if not shared or diagnosed by the right people.

Before training the body, it's vital to be able to channel and learn how to train the mind. The mind can be the most powerful tool as it facilitates what the body does. The brain plays an integral role in how the body follows. My question is, how hard is it to channel the mind to allow the body to follow? Some of the most famous human beings have been successful due to their ability to be strong mentally to overcome adversity. I must admit I still battle at times to get my mind right, which is human, but I truly believe it's part of our own development to achieve what we were set out to do.

The truth is, sometimes this can be a lot deeper than just your current environment. This could be something that has stemmed from childhood. Mental health is slowly being accepted in modern society, and more people are slowly accepting help. It is something that has changed my whole scope on listening and understanding mankind. For those who don't know, for a while I had suffered silently from it, rebounding my thoughts and feelings as something I just needed to fix internally and sort out myself. This, at times, affected my closest and dearest to whom I owe the world for tolerating me and helping me overcome it. The truth is, there is no shame in getting help or reaching out to be heard. I struggled a lot, screaming inside for help, but didn't want to burden others with my issues, and often watered down or dimmed down the pain.

The problem is that didn't solve anything but merely delayed the symptoms, piling on the stress. I lost some important people in my life, lost my dream business ambition that I had left home to set up, and was fortunate to survive a life-threatening car accident, which today makes me count every blessing I have. I questioned many things, and for someone spiritual, my faith was tested more than I can imagine, and left me contemplating life and my purpose.

People struggling with mental health could be in your family, living next door, teaching your children, working in the desk next to you in the office, or serving you at a restaurant. Although the general perception of mental illness has improved over the past decade, studies show the stigma against mental illness is still powerful—largely due to media stereotypes and lack of education. People tend to attach negative stigmas to mental health conditions at a far higher rate than to other diseases and disabilities such as cancer and heart disease. In the United Kingdom, one in four people experience mental health problems such as anxiety, depression, loss of a loved one, or financial problems.

How do we help spread awareness when it's a silent killer? We promote being a better version of ourselves by showing individuals respect and acceptance regardless of their status or position in our communities. This helps remove a significant barrier for them to successfully cope with their illness. Having people see you as an individual and not as your illness can make a big difference for someone who is struggling with their health.

Things to remember when going through tough times:

1. Everything can and will change.
2. You have overcome challenges before and will continue to do so.
3. In every lesson is a blessing.
4. Your calling is far greater than you know, and by staying true to what you believe in, good things will come.
5. Take things lightly, and when not sure, take more time to respond.
6. Being kind to yourself is the best medicine.
7. Yesterday didn't go as planned; few more hours to go and we can reset that and begin a different page.
8. Reset your emotions through meditation, prayer, or just faith.
9. Don't focus on what you don't have; be thankful for what you do, and try to increase your list by adding something every day.
10. Find your peace, and everything will fall in place.
11. Giving back can give you a lot when you don't expect it.

I often relate my life to sport, so when reading the term *sport*, substitute the term for *life*, so you can visualize it. One of the most overused clichés in sport is that 90 percent of performance is mental. In my opinion, the problem is that 90 percent of coaches and athletes spend 100 percent of their time working on the physical aspect rather than acknowledging the magnitude of mental training. Metaphorically it's vital that we strike the right balance to be able to perform our daily objectives to their highest potential. Sports science has offered us some wonderful insights on performance and physical attributes evolving in the game. I've noticed that a lot of questions are generally asked about mind-set when athletes face challenges, which shows its importance. The great comebacks in world sport after losing a final or a fight to overcome the odds has always been a story we all love to hear.

Setting high yet realistic goals can aid a long way when setting a plan. Anthony Robbins often discussed massive action plan (MAP) as key when setting personal goals. What I love about that is that setting MASSIVE plans often results in your lowest being average and your highest being amazing and fulfilling.

Here are a few tips for mental training:

1. Draw out a MAP (I actually enjoy using paper for this despite digital being available in all formats).
2. Set high yet realistic goals (print it for the day/month/year, log it, and review it).

3. Set a realistic time frame to be able to execute it (however short or long, it still sets you an objective).

4. Reward yourself throughout the time frame to promote enjoying the process.

5. Use mental imagery. Remember, the mind is your best muscle. "Big arms can move rocks but words can move mountains," said Rocky Balboa.

6. Take photos to also enhance visuals in goal setting (whether on your phone or tablet, create a folder to go back to and look at).

7. Manage anxiety effectively by planning realistic outcomes (focus on journey and not just result).

8. Practice gratitude (take an hour a week to start to show gratitude by visiting a charity or shelter).

9. Give yourself the same advice you'd give a trusted family member or dear friend (we often give the best advice when we aren't involved).

10. Create a healthy mind-set (find what helps you in your situation with your preferences without worrying about anyone else) to be happy.

11. The rule of reciprocation—this is the idea of you giving, and later, the universe giving back to you.

12. Hold yourself accountable (the world doesn't owe you anything so instead of expecting, give to the world and it will all come back in due time).

13. One percent every day goes a long way.

Visualization
I struggled at times when I wasn't able to visualize what it was that I wanted to achieve. Being honest with myself about what my objective was, and identifying what I wanted to get out of the situation was difficult when being general. Stripping down to asking myself, what is it that makes me happy? What am I driven by? Is it money? Fame? Family? Status? Which of those last? Long enough to be able to maintain happiness. How would you put those in order of importance to you?

1. Fame
2. Family
3. Status
4. Money
5. Love
6. Other

The answer to the above for me was family, and being able to support them with love and anything else they needed. Rather than focusing on what you don't have, appreciate and value what you do, and things can go a long way.

I've always been fascinated with creative minds and how the brain functions with those who don't follow the trend and create their own path, as "crazy" or as outrageous as their ideas may appear. I then strip it back and visualize how their brain worked and func-tioned during their journey. It definitely adds a whole demographic of mind-set and thought process when analyzing an action or experience. I want to end the chapter with a quote from Bruce Lee, "Empty your mind, and be formless, shapeless, like water. If you put water into a cup, it becomes the cup. You put water into a bottle and it becomes the bottle."

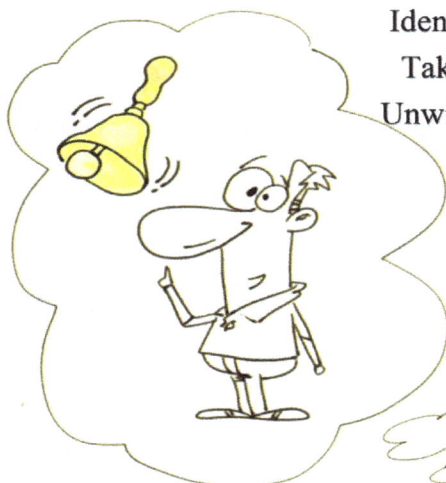

Identify Your Key
Takeaways from
Unwind Your Mind

❖ Takeaway 1

❖ Takeaway 2

❖ Takeaway 3

❖ Takeaway 4

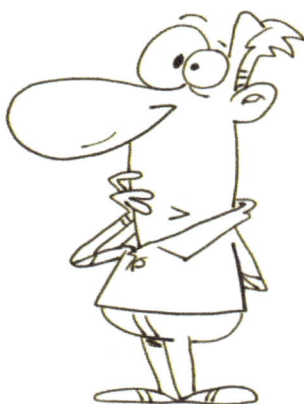

DOMINO 3: Train Smart, Not Hard

Food is the most widely abused anti-anxiety drug, and exercise is the most potent yet underutilized antidepressant.

—Billy Phillips

Domino 3:

Training

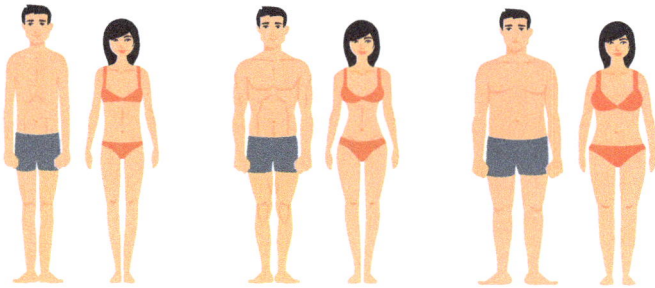

Ectomorph   Mesomorph   Endomorph

BEFORE ENTERING THE world of training, we strip it down and tend to look at ourselves in the mirror. Have you ever asked yourself what body type are you? How does your body adapt to different styles of training?

There are three basic human body types: the endomorph, the mesomorph, and the ectomorph. Despite a lot of factors coming into play, such as genetics, medical history, and environment, these give you a good baseline to measure which category you fall under. Within time and consistency, you may also find your body type shifting from mesomorph to endomorph, for example. We demonstrated earlier the different ways to fuel the three body types, but what are their individual symptoms when categorizing them?

Ectomorph
Ectomorphs, known in some respect as "hard gainers," often struggle to gain weight or muscle and have a thin frame. They tend to have a lean body with long limbs, and even when they gain weight, it's barely recognizable unless they reveal their upper body in their swimsuits. The way you look under this body type doesn't necessarily mean you are weak; you could be extremely strong when training the body through recorded progressive training. However, be ready to complement your training with the right fuel because it is equally important to make those gains.

Mesomorph
Mesomorphs tend to have wide shoulders, a more rounded frame with a relatively moderate joint structure. One thing we have to be very mindful of is that in this body type you can't get away with eating whatever you want, especially as age catches up. However, because you have a good starting base it does help in regaining fitness or resetting your body into peak mode if you don't fall off-track for a short period. Don't neglect your cardio or interval training

from time to time to maintain or sculpt what you have.

Endomorph
Endomorphs, when gaining weight, tend to face the most difficulty if they are not careful in losing it instantly. Their build is a little wider than an ectomorph or mesomorph, with a thick ribcage, wide hips, and shorter limbs. The common issue faced in this body type is that gaining weight is often a combination of muscle and fat, emphasizing the fuel and nutrition even more than any of the other body types. The art lies in being wiser, accepting what base you have but finding the right balance to what makes you feel good as well as look good.

How do we train? Weights, cardio, yoga, circuit training, Barry's Bootcamp, Orangetheory Fitness, or animal flow. Keep the following questions in mind when thinking about your training regime:

1. What works for you?
2. How long have you been doing it for?
3. Have you seen results?
4. Is it purely aesthetic or performance based?
5. At what point do we switch it up?

Let's take things in perspective. When a baby is born, there is something very special about its movement. The baby is born with freedom of movement, flexibility, and mobility. How does that change when we get older?

Habit of movement
Habit of lifestyle
Habit of range of motion

Now despite strength obviously being a factor, which can be developed at a young age, I often find myself admiring the way they move. The excitement of the next step and the vulnerability of standing up again when falling is a joy. How can we promote exercise at a young age without stunting growth? Gymnastics, swimming, body weight, yoga, calisthenics, and parkour spring to mind.

Here's my theory. No one was born an adult, so everyone has a child in them. Practicing those disciplines promote all those amazing attributes we described in the beginning of this chapter. Now that's not saying weight training doesn't work, because I believe that performing weight training, especially with compound movements, is extremely beneficial. Some of the best results I have personally experienced are when I used a combination of weight training and high-intensity interval training. When referring to weight training, it doesn't mean lift as heavy as you can with no purpose. It means that once you master your own body weight in different planes and motions, then you can progress to going heavier. Some of the hardest styles of training I have encountered were mastering body weight in movements I wasn't used to, which really exposed my imbalances.

Those resulted in strengthening areas such as the core and trunk, to be able to move and function a lot better. Unfortunately, to keep up with trends and times we rush ourselves—whether it's pressure to keep up or set the bar high with workouts. The fact is, science hasn't changed, so no matter what's trending, the human body works the same way it did 1,000 years ago. Yes, we are spoilt with new technology and incredible applications, which are there to assist but not there to take over your world! Gary Vee said it best, "It's a game about being best and not being first! Everyone's trying to catch that next best thing without focusing on the current." The reason why he's so successful is that "he's best at executing the current." Bruce Lee agreed with this and strongly promoted it through his martial arts and lifestyle: "I fear not the man who has practiced 10,000 kicks once, but I fear the man who has practiced one kick 10,000 times."

I feel we ignore the boring things, such as correctives and basic movement, to focus on the "cool" workouts. This results in injury and a lot of money spent on rectifying wrong movements that we didn't even know we were doing.

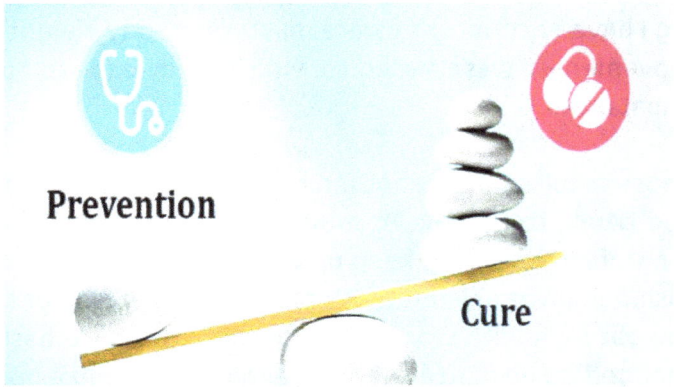

Prevention

Cure

How Often Shall I Train? And for How Long?

The body is a complicated machine. As discussed earlier on how to fuel your body, it influences the mechanics of it. Fitness is a relationship. You can't cheat on it, take shortcuts, and expect it to work. Training four hours a day may not be what is required for your body to achieve results. Using the machine for four hours a day in the long term may not be beneficial because it requires recovery and maintenance. Try between 40 to 60 minutes of efficient training, and you would be amazed at how much time you could save. Doing so doesn't mean you have to rush the exercise because you only have 40 minutes. Tension training can also be done here where the focus is on the actual muscle through the move by pausing or holding the action. This enables you to feel the muscle more when executing the exercise.

Let's take a familiar exercise like the push-up, for example. Take four seconds to go down, pause for two at the bottom, and take one second to come up. Now repeat that ten times. Compare that to ten standard push-ups, and you're more likely to feel it. This can be done with most body weight moves. A lot of the time we become more efficient when we tune our mind to our muscle. This promotes the likelihood of more successful results as you aim to reach physical and mental goals. It also helps sharpen our cognitive ability to become sharper and more alert.

Now that's not to say you can't achieve great things by dedicating more or less than that, but I found this method successful when trying to reach my optimal physical performance. I've always been asked the million-dollar question followed by the half-a-million-dollar question. How do I lose weight? And what's the best program I can do to train? And honestly, before that, I ask the question: What are you currently doing? Are you mixing it up and adding variety to your workout? Because I truly believe that variety = sustain-ability = longevity, because you are feeding the body so much knowledge and education on what works for your body. Why does our training, gym membership, or motivation drop after a while?

I consider it a privilege when people allow me to assist them with their goals. There is something about being able to achieve results with someone, especially when they have trusted you with something, they haven't been able to master yet. A lot of these people under-stand exercise and how to eat moderate portions, but sometimes don't realize their true potential or how close they are to achieving something that can change their lifestyle on a daily basis, bringing happiness. I learned from a lot of masters around the world who stood out for many reasons. The reasons include the following:

1. Knowledge with years and years of study
2. Experience of dealing with several clients with a variety of different cases
3. Delivery that was equally as important because there is no point having all the knowledge in the world if you can't deliver that to help people

All of the above have inspired me to be very mindful of that when listening to clients and in solving their challenges.

The secret formula to losing weight is **discipline!**

Now, as basic and obvious as that answer is, regardless of whatever trends or super pills that are out there, there are no corners that can be cut. As highlighted in this book, a lot comes down to mind-set and creating your own environment to be able to eliminate false conclusions. Let me put it this way. Start your own blank canvas, and give it time to flourish. It's easier and, quite frankly, more exciting to be able to experience your own journey and then to go by what worked for someone else (hence the canvas analogy). Be realistic with time. As humans, we often just get bored, make excuses, and jump on the next hype train. If it's taken you longer than expected to get back into routine and you aren't happy with where you are, allow yourself the time to get back on track and be strong with your planning and discipline through all the dominos discussed in the book.

HIIT Training
High-intensity interval training (HIIT) involves short bursts of training that elevate the heart rate, followed by short active recovery periods. The pros are time efficiency, challenge, and effectiveness. HIIT cannot be done every day, as the body requires a sufficient amount of energy to perform it effectively at the highest level, and not all age groups enjoy the strain on the

body. There are ways of working around it, especially if you have a coach who can measure according to the individual. With this comes EPOC (excess postexercise oxygen consumption), which is what happens to the body after you work out, resulting in your metabolism speeding up. EPOC also promotes burning more calories as the body adjusts to returning to its default levels, which can go up to 48 hours from your workout. One of my coaches (shout out Coach Randy) in Thailand told me a long time ago, "It's not always what you do in the session that is outstanding, it's what it sets you up for the next 48 hours."

I particularly enjoyed the Japanese Protocol Tabata, which was a simple formula you could use with any exercises to create a challenge in a short period of time. Now when performed at full effort, it can be incredibly challenging for the body. Factors such as breathing help you endure the duration of the Tabata promoting endurance and stamina due to the short rest periods.

Here's one of my favorites: 20 seconds on, 10 seconds off recovery x 8 reps.

What I like to do is switch it up, so I might do the first four the same and the second four something different.

1. 20 seconds on the assault bike
2. 10 seconds recovery x 4
3. 20 seconds of sprints
4. 10 seconds of rest x 4

You can substitute the exercises for any exercises you find challenging or want to improve on, but remember to challenge yourself and use the recovery period to reset, and then go again. This is just an example of HIIT training that I personally have seen a lot of results with and that you can modify.

LISS Training

Low-intensity steady state (LISS) cardio is a form of exercise that involves less impact and a slower approach to training levels. Walking at a steady pace on an incline for a longer period of time is also effective to stay active between tough workout days. I often saw a lot of bodybuilders who monitored their weight before competitions used this to regulate their calories. There is usually a debate on which is better for fat loss and how often to do either. I honestly believe that they complement each other greatly.

Here's my thought on combining the two styles.

On Sunday I would create a (HIIT) session that had a combination of weights and sprints. The body would require a lot of energy, which means my body would be burning for up to 48 hours.

On Monday I wouldn't want to miss a day of training when I still had fuel in the engine but didn't want to exhaust myself to the point I would be out for a few days, so I would either go for a walk (LISS), which would be an active recovery session, or go cycling.

Tuesday, I would play 8 aside football for an hour.

Wednesday, I would take a day off to rest with maybe some movement in the pool as my active recovery day, or just laze about by the pool and catch some sun.

Thursday, I would box for 12 rounds at 3 minutes a round with a minute's break, either on the bag or have a coach hold the mitts for me.

Friday, I would do LISS workout.

Saturday, I would see how I felt assessing the week and listening to my body. If I needed the rest, I would rest, and if not, I would decide which of the above I would like to do that day.

Remember that a lot of the factors that affect my week are how much water I drank, how I slept, how many hours I worked, whether my nutrition went as per plan. This may vary from week to week, especially when you skip a day or two and you feel guilty. All that this means is that you are creating a positive habit that is part of your lifestyle and the body wants more!

How Do I Know If I'm Doing HIIT or LISS?

If, like me, you need to see numbers and get motivated by setting personal goals, invest in a heart rate monitor that syncs to your personal device and that you can always revert to and keep track of. With modern technology, there are some fantastic apps and devices out there that keep track of weekly, monthly, and yearly goals. This has helped me a lot in setting goals and breaking personal records even when no one is looking!

Here's a formula:

220 - age = Max heart rate

220 - 28=192

60% of 192 = 115.2
70% of 192 = 134.4
80% of 192 = 153.6

Weight Loss Tip
When staying between 60 and 80 percent of your maximum heart rate, you are burning fat specifically.

When going over 80 percent, you are improving your endurance and stamina, increasing your fitness levels.

What does efficient training consist of? Less of breaks, socializing, and spending time on Instagram! Dedicate that time to yourself, and use it as "me time" to make you feel better.

How Do We Feel Better?
Depending on your respective fitness level, training is something to help the body, not deplete it. I recently read some very interesting methods by Feras Zahabi who is an incredible coach in the mixed martial arts world—training some of the best athletes. GSP, George St-Pierre, is one of the best examples not just in sport but in life on how you should look after your body. At age 38, he portrays a body of health intrinsically and extrinsically. Having achieved all he can in the sport of mixed martial arts by winning multiple world titles and accolades, he's been managed very well by his coach Zahabi, who believes in "flow training." I agree with his beliefs that the human body functions at a certain rate, and there's no way around it as it depends on several factors individually. The idea is to train smart and efficiently to accumulate the right

"minutes" under your belt in order to achieve optimal performance.

Stress, Recovery, and Adaptation

Something I have personally experienced and tried is flow training, which is training at 60–70 percent five times a week rather than twice a week at 100 percent. His philosophy is, with training at 100 percent comes soreness, which is being in a zone that could be detrimental to your long-term goal, risking injury. When looking at progress at the end of the year, 60–70 percent would enable you to have achieved more volume. I found this very interesting and definitely worth experimenting with the body.

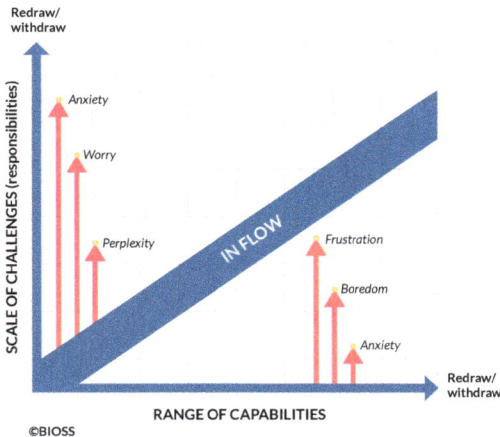

Adapted from Csikszentmihalyi, M. Optical Experience
Cambridge Univeristy Press 1988

Proposed by Mihály Csíkszentmihályi in the Positive Psychology, *flow* is the mental state in which a person in an activity is fully immersed in a feeling of energized focus, full involvement, and success in the process of the activity. According to Csíkszentmihályi, flow is completely focused motivation. It is a single-minded immersion and represents perhaps the ultimate in harnessing the emotions in the service of performing and learning. In flow, the emotions are not just contained and channeled but also positive, energized, and aligned with the task at hand. Mihály Csíkszentmihályi said, "The best moments in our lives are not the passive, receptive, relaxing times. The best moments usually occur if a person's body or mind is stretched to its limits in a voluntary effort to accomplish something difficult and worthwhile."

When Michael Jordan or Mohammed Ali were in the zone, they weren't overthinking how they are going to make the right pass or throw the perfect punch, because that would interrupt their state of mind and throw them off. Through practice and repetition, the body was programmed to execute the correct movements, which didn't require them to think but merely act on all the hard work and time that already had been put in the gym. Absorption in a task indicates the absence of the self and a merging of your awareness into the activity you are engaged in. Training at volume and actually having a periodization plan promotes longevity without burning yourself out.

I grew up in an environment where one believed that if you train hard, then you can enjoy the competition. It did work for me, but eventually, as time passed, my body took a beating, and I could feel my joints suffering from the wear and tear. After suffering multiple injuries, I was forced to study and learn more about how I could rectify that, and, if I could go back to a younger me, what would I do differently? In conclusion, the older I got, the smarter I had to be to achieve results because the body functions a lot more different with the experiences we accumulate over the years.

The sooner we decide to disconnect from our ego and find a solution for every obstacle, the sooner we achieve great results! We all face setbacks and injuries along the way—it's the way we switch our mental mode on to adhere to our physical needs. Having experienced my own battles with injuries, it helped me understand the true mind-set of what my athletes face and what is required to highlight and focus on throughout the different stages of rehab. It opens the opportunity for you to understand and focus on other skills we can develop, which we might have been neglecting.

We often neglect prevention skills because it is usually under the idea that there's no point in wasting time if I'm ok. The problem with that statement is that unfortunately, it takes something bad to make us think how we can cure it rather than preventing it in the first place. How many of us get sick or injured because we didn't see something coming and then wonder how it happened? The human anatomy is complex and not something we can always visually see, so if the body is beginning to react a certain way, our common response is, it's not that serious or that bad. This isn't only relevant to training but is equally important with your immune system. The positive factor is that the value of health and fitness in modern society is getting the attention it deserves and the awareness from a very young age. This means that it is being taught at schools. When visiting schools and speaking to the children and parents at seminars and events, I was so impressed with how much they were aware and educated on the matter from such a young age.

Tim Ferris described it best, "Pursuing rapid increase in performance without doing 'pre-hab' for injury prevention is like getting in an F-1 racing car without checking the tires." Perhaps the world's most in-demand injury prevention specialist was Gray Cook, who was a huge influence on the NFL, MLB, NHL, and NBA. His philosophy was that the most likely cause of injury was neither weakness nor tightness but imbalance in the body. He highlighted cases when despite clients believing it was one factor, it was lack of movement in the hips; predominantly one side more than the other would hinder performance, and that would eventually cause injury. Now, why is that relevant to a normal person like me?

Gray's brainchild and fundamental tool for identifying imbalances was the functional movement screen (FMS). FMS identifies movement asymmetries or deficiencies that prevent athletes from injuries. Now how is that relevant to us? Because we always promote the thought of balancing a healthy lifestyle but the problem is that we sometimes don't know how to measure that. FMS is a series of seven movement tests, which is often scored on a three-point scale by a certified professional. It's designed to identify two things: asymmetry (left to right imbalances) and wobbling and shifting (motor control issues). Now I'm trying to simplify this as much as possible so I don't ramble on about FMS.

Here are the seven movements:

1. Deep squat
2. Hurdle step
3. In-line lunge
4. Active straight leg raise
5. Shoulder mobility
6. Rotary stability
7. Trunk stability push-up

To learn more about FMS, I would recommend checking out https://www.functionalmovement.com/system/fms.

Corrective Exercise

Corrective exercise helps in enhancing efficiency and performance levels; it reduces the risk of injury and allows the body to rehabilitate in the best way from injury. The benefits from correctives enhance the quality of life due to movements that are easier and less stressful. I loved Paul Cheks's analogy, "The basic movement patterns are like the 0–9 keys on a calculator. All other numbers are still combinations of the basics." That was something I noticed with trends in the health and fitness industry. How someone could start on intermediate even if they hadn't mastered the beginner movements and patterns, especially in classes. When Gray Cook was asked for four corrective exercises to fix the most common weaknesses, here's what he recommended:

1. Chop and lift
2. Turkish get up (my favorite)
3. Two-arm, single-leg deadlift
4. Cross-body, one-arm, single-leg deadlift

There's no rush to do them all at the same time as you may choose to focus on one before moving to the second. It is harder to visualize the exercises from text rather than videos, so if you're not sure, ask a professional about form and technique. These movements are to build a strong foundation to help us function better mechanically and get that strong and healthy balance for everyday life. The use of foam rollers, resistance bands, and even monitors is now being incorporated before competition to prepare the body to perform at its maximum capacity. The hard work is often done with the physios, trainers, or medical staff before, but these certainly help warm the body up.

Mobility
Mobility refers to our ability to move freely without stress on the body. Our flexibility is dependent on the range of motion of our muscles. Good mobility can assist your flexibility and vice versa. The body is put through different stages throughout the day, so being consistent with mobility enables the muscles to recognize being functional quicker and reduces risk of injury through muscle memory. I try not to get caught up in what I read in the magazines but go back to the principles of training. In the modern fitness world, we are trending over different forms of exercises weekly! The point is, if you want to be stronger or faster in a desired skill, then dedicate your time to perfecting the total package. A simple example is running:

Why does a marathon runner look different physically in comparison to a sprinter? They train differently in their respective skills to enhance performance, so despite being in the same sport, they train, eat, recover, and replenish in a completely different way.

So, we take from this chapter that training in a way that works for your friend may not work for you because we have all different backgrounds, histories, medical conditions, and strengths and weaknesses. Don't be scared to see a specialist for something that you require further knowledge on. The human anatomy is worth investing time on because it will help you function and perform better in everyday life. Training doesn't have to be four hours a day. HIIT or Tabata (Japanese Protocol) can get you the same results in shorter workout periods, giving you exactly the same results with more time to spend with the family or friends.

Your body needs servicing like a car, so look after it by incorporating mobility, corrective exercise, fuel, and recovery. If it helps to write programs down before you train, then do so as it promotes progress, planning, and organization. It also works very well with striving to do better in the long run and not being stuck on the same weight, speed, or goal. Training in different regions exposed me to different methods all around the world. What fascinates me is not necessarily the facility as much as the person I'm going to meet. Despite attaining a degree in the field, had I not approached these professionals with an open mind, I would have missed out on a wealth of knowledge and techniques. A lot of times in this book I interlink the dominos, which shows how vital it is to appreciate and value each pillar because holistically they merge to function fluently, with no restrictions.

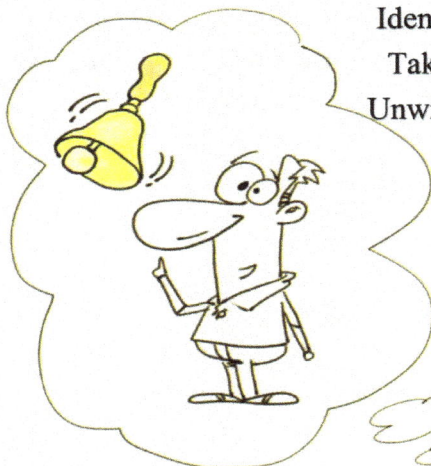

Identify Your Key
Takeaways from
Unwind Your Mind

❖ Takeaway 1

❖ Takeaway 2

❖ Takeaway 3

❖ Takeaway 4

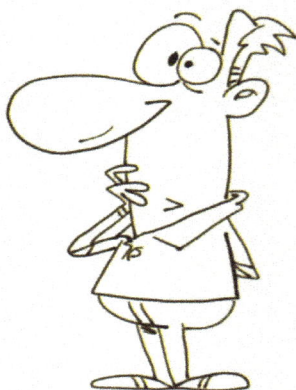

Domino 4: Resetting Your Environment

You can't make positive choices for the rest of your life, without an environment that makes those choices easy, natural, and enjoyable.

—Deepak Chopra

Domino 4:

Resetting Your Environment

I'VE OFTEN HEARD the phrase, "I've got to get away," and my question straight back is, away from what? What is it that you are finding challenging? Challenges are part of everyday life and this is no different. I've been fortunate to have traveled to camps around the world to experience different approaches to physical and mental goals. It's costly and can have an adverse effect when you return back to the root problem.

Don't get me wrong; it's worked for me when I have traveled to get away and get a little peace of mind at times, but looking back, we create our own environment by eliminating or introducing factors. What if I could reset my environment without traveling? Make minor adjustments to help me with productivity, be better with the family, or just enjoy the simple things more. I do understand that life can be a hundred miles an hour at times, and there are things that are out of our hands. If you're like me and don't like change, then it's hard to get out of routine or something you are used to. I lived in the same house for twenty-four years before moving countries, which set the route of my comfort zone. Dubai was the destination in which I learnt a lot about myself by facing what everyone faces when they move to a completely different environment. The fact that you learn fast if you don't already know what it is like to live alone makes you appreciate the building blocks our families set for us when we are growing up.

I once heard someone referring to habits as patterns, which really resonated with me when I was growing up. We have patterns of actions of how we work, eat, and relate to other people. Some of these patterns are healthy and positive for our personal growth and development, and some are toxic—it takes time for us to realize the effects. Has that started to get you thinking about your own habits and behavior patterns? It takes twenty-one days to create a habit, and ninety-two days to incorporate a lifestyle change. If you had three things you would like to improve on, what would they be?

1_____

2_____

3_____

List them down, and monitor them over the next three weeks, choosing a day per week as a deadline to monitor progress. That's why I have attached a gratitude journal later on, which really helps balance my equilibrium when tackling a feeling or thought that crosses my mind. It helps me put things in perspective and allows me to stay grateful for things we often neglect. Learn to appreciate and love yourself because without that I truly believe we cannot love others unconditionally. As obvious as that sounds, I wasn't able to fully commit blindly for a long time because I wasn't content with what I had to offer. Bill Phillips said, "Focus on progress not perfection," because if you cannot overcome feelings of self-doubt, it doesn't matter how much accurate information about training or nutrition you have. This doesn't only affect you but also those in your circle or environment who are around you. Now, this doesn't only work one way—you gravitate more people to you with good healthy energy in case you needed another reason. Energy can be such a beautiful thing that is contagious when you take time to reflect and appreciate it.

One of the most beautiful things I came across was the universal law of reciprocation—I came across it in 1999 but didn't really understand its true meaning until I applied it much later. I coached a university women's football team in the Middle East that I was introduced to when I first moved to the United Arab Emirates, which was pure coincidence. That role at American University Dubai (AUD) could have been handed to anyone, but following the rule of timing and being in the right place at the right time, I was offered it and I accepted. Eventually, I took charge of this team and took them under my wing, independently coaching them for free for years for the love of the sport. It didn't make financial sense at the time, especially because I was away from home and needed to work to support myself.

However, unconsciously, I was following the rule of reciprocation—the best way to receive it is to give it. Obviously, we all have bad days, which raises questions on why we do things when others don't. Many people want to get before they give, and I'm sure we have all been there at some point or another in our lives. Regardless of my personal issues at the time, the way I looked at coaching was as a form of escapism. To do something I love unconditionally and to be away from my phone and computer for the hours spent with that team was incredible. This applied to me in so many ways when I look back at my career as a trainer and a coach. When I focused on creating value for others, I may have not seen something instantly, but later it came in many forms of satisfaction, acknowledgment, fulfillment, self-esteem, and friendship.

Five years later I was acknowledged as Sport 360 Coach of the Year in the UAE for my contribution to developing women's football in the community. I share this because you don't have to be from a certain religion or culture to be able to apply this, but believe that by giving you receive; the universe honestly has a plan for you when you are doing good for others. When looking at ourselves, we tend to ignore small factors that could contribute to big changes in the long run.

Let's consider space and entering a space; if we leave it a certain way when we are experiencing an emotion, the next time we enter it, we will feel the same energy we felt when we left it. The purpose of resetting each room is not simply to clean up after the last action but to prepare for the next action. This does link with planning and preparation and being disciplined enough to execute the next step in the right direction. Whenever you organize a space for its intended purpose, you are preparing it to make the next action easy. This is one of the most practical and simple ways to improve your habits. Setting up your next few steps can come a long way, especially when it becomes habitual.

Declutter
Remove unnecessary items from an untidy or overcrowded place. Now visualize decluttering your mind, which, let's face it, if you're like me, can be messy at

times. Just like our cabinets and cupboards, our minds need tidying up from time to time. That all comes from the environment we set and how we handle certain situations. Getting rid of all that nonessential mental baggage is crucial to stay focused, motivated, and productive.

Key Takeaways

1. Leave something the way you would like to pick up from it.
2. Hold yourself accountable in the moment.
3. Set priorities.
4. Learn to let go and not dwell.
5. Give what you're doing the attention it requires.
6. Breathe.
7. Learn to take a timeout to reset.
8. Do some coloring or painting.
9. Empty out the fridge.
10. Do some volunteer work.
11. Spend time with children or pets.
12. Visit a place you were at some time ago and reflect on how far you have come.
13. Apologize.

When it comes to resetting your environment, it all starts intrinsically and how you feel inside. When you treat yourself the way you want others to treat you, then many factors are at peace. However, if you don't, how do you expect anyone else to enjoy your company. That's why it starts with you and how you look after yourself—how you fuel, rest, recover, love, support, be happy for others and give! In the world we live in, it's easy to get caught up in distracting factors such as social media or politics at work. A lot of us get caught up and focus on what we don't have rather than what we do. Expect adversity and be prepared to transform obstacles into energy. Harness the power of positive pressure by embracing challenges. Reset your environment.

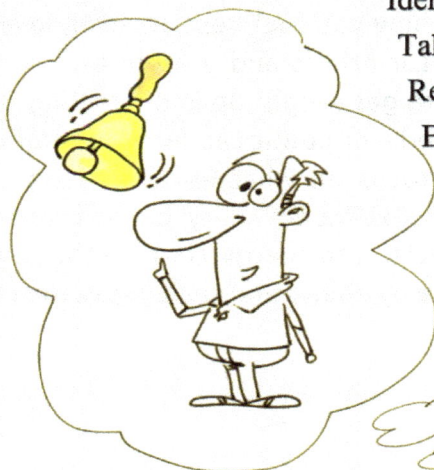

Identify Your Key
Takeaways from
Resetting Your
Environment

❖ Takeaway 1

❖ Takeaway 2

❖ Takeaway 3

❖ Takeaway 4

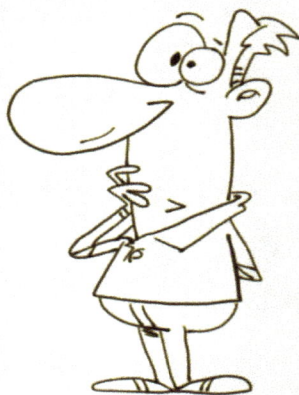

DOMINO 5: Recovery— Important Enough to Dedicate a Chapter to It

Prevention is better than cure.

—Desiderius Erasmus

Domino 5:

Recovery

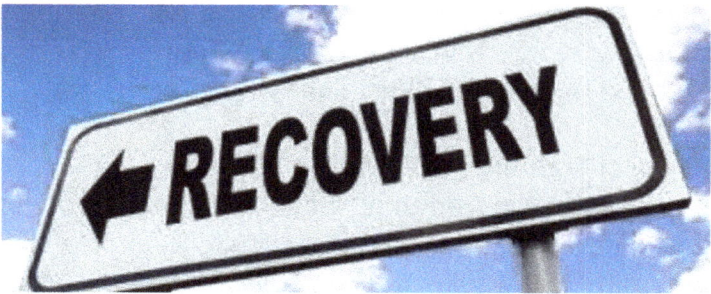

I COULDN'T HELP write a book on mental and physical health without including a domino that is probably the most neglected in balancing goal setting. I would even go as far as saying too much training can hinder longevity goals without the right balance of recovery. How so? You could be straining the mind or body in ways that result to injury or anxiety, which is completely against being happy or feeling great within yourself. That's why as I mentioned in Pillar 3: flow training made so much sense. I must admit I have fallen guilty of overtraining many times in the past but this is where the readers can hopefully avoid the mistakes I made and do better.

I tore my cruciate ligament playing football without knowing it had previously been a minor injury I picked up with one sudden turn—it had kept me out for seven months. Obviously, injuries can happen to anyone at any given time, but as mentioned in the book, with the right corrective measures and fuel, it can reduce the chances massively. Allowing the body to reset and adjust to whatever you're planning to put it through next is worth putting in perspective. There are factors we need to consider when highlighting recovery:

Physical Training
Approaching the "red zone" when your body is close to breaking, but you want to finish off the week on a high before the big weekend. The body is allowed to adapt to the stress associated with exercise, replenishing muscle glycogen (energy stores), and providing time for the body tissue to repair.

Psychological Stress
Stress and anxiety from work, home, or even family could take its toll when trying to manage the above and more.

Health
If you catch a virus or get ill when your immune system is deteriorating and you're fighting to recover from an infection.

Environment
Recover from your environment or adjust to a new climate, workspace, or crowd of people.

I was always asked how you know when it's too much. Quite frankly, the answer is how you feel. Monitoring your goals and achievements can be awesome, and it can also indicate where you are at. However, we are not programmed the same and don't always produce the same outcome. Meaning you could achieve a great month of training and productivity this month feeling satiated and great. If you're good to match that next month for results, that's fine, but if not, tackle the third consecutive month bearing in mind you allowed the body and mind to progress to be stress-free in month two. The only issue sometimes is because I believe they all go hand in hand. We change the way we eat because of the way we train; that also affects the way we rest, so as long as you can manage the above, then I believe 4/5 is not considered a setback but a step forward in tackling the year. I monitor and keep track of this by having a heart-rate monitor and application synced to my phone. This helps me set individual goals for the year as I get quite competitive and work better when I have something to achieve.

Here are a few tips to help with this chapter:

1. Trigger point therapy or myofascial release can be done through foam rolling before or after training or even on a daily basis. It promotes correcting muscle imbalances, improving range of motion, and speeding up recovery by helping with blood circulation.

2. Foam rollers are now extremely common and easy to carry around especially when not having the luxury of getting a massage whenever needed.

3. Being able to dedicate time for yourself in the world we live in isn't too much to ask, is it? With social media around and the technology available to us, our brain works at 200 mph. Meditation helps channel and bring everything to the surface. Closing your eyes, relaxing your body, and channeling your breathing a few minutes a day can really help.

4. Guided meditation for self-healing can be found through YouTube or online platforms. Being able to reset the brain and mind helps manifest into the rest of your day controlling anxiety, enhancing self-awareness, and lengthening attention spans.

5. Salt baths can prove beneficial. In water, it breaks down into magnesium and sulfate. Mixed martial artists normally use this to cut weight or relaxing joints after a hard training session. I recommend picking up some real Epsom salts from the pharmacy, which would really help. Soak for ten to fifteen minutes whether you use ice for an ice bath or heat for a good hot bath.

6. Cold water immersion can stimulate blood flow and really make a difference when incorporating it in your lifestyle especially at the start of the day before you head out to work. Some of the most phenomenal athletes and successful people have attributed their recovery and routine to it. Cold showers and cryo chambers have been extremely successful and beneficial in enhancing performance and longevity. This helps reduce swelling and inflammation lowering the damaged tissues temperature and constricting the blood vessels.

7. Getting a massage helps release scar tissue and reduces inflammation and soreness. It also helps with blood circulation and improves the immune system. There are many forms and massage techniques, but my personal preference is a deep-tissue sports massage by a qualified professional who understands the human anatomy.

8. Water plays a significant role in the process of recovery—from helping digest vital nutrients to repairing muscles damaged during exercise. Your body depends on water to survive. Every cell, tissue, and organ in your body needs water to work properly. For example, your body uses water to maintain its temperature, remove waste, and lubricate your joints. I invested in one of those liter temperature bottles that helped me keep a good count of how many liters I consume a day, especially when working or moving from job to job. If it wasn't finished by about 8 pm, I knew I was slacking or not up to par for my hydration for the day. There are ways of monitoring that personally and that is through the color of urine:

HYDRATED

HYDRATED

HYDRATED

MILDLY DEHYDRATED

MODERATELY DEHYDRATED

MODERATELY HYDRATED

DEHYDRATED

SEVERELY DEHYDRATED

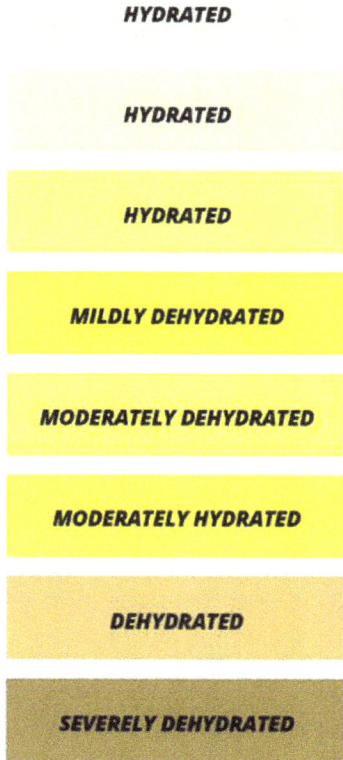

9. Sleep enhances muscle recovery through pro-
    tein synthesis and human growth hormone
    release. Sleep has a profound effect on muscle
    growth and physical well-being. Sleeping six to
    eight hours is ideal bearing in mind that your
    body and brain shut off completely from the

world. Some may attempt to sleep for eight hours but actually only get five to six due to their brain overthinking or analyzing the day's events in bed. That's why it's not recommended to be staring at a screen before you go to bed whether its phone, computer, or TV. Invest in some blue light glasses if you have issues sleeping due to staring at screens all day.

The recovery process also ties in with the environment, which was mentioned earlier in this book; it really does make a difference. Having a clean space that isn't decluttered helps settle the brain before going to bed, which does relax the mind. Whether you're into scents, smells, or remedies, I found it extremely helpful when going to bed if the sheets were clean, the room was at the right temperature, and the smell was great. These are all minor adjustments that really made a big difference in the long run when trying to fix my sleep. When you don't sleep enough, cortisol levels rise, which activate reward centers in your brain and make you crave food. You also produce more ghrelin (known as the hunger hormone), resulting in you feeling hungrier more often. That would explain the urge for reaching out for late-night snacks, foods with sugar, and salty bites.

In Chinese philosophy, they believe that the window from 11 pm to 3 am is the time in which the body (gall bladder) is at its most powerful to sleep. Missing that bracket messes with your system and carries over into the following day. Having visited and researched into a lot of ancient Chinese health philosophy, I was intrigued by how they managed to maintain such a balanced lifestyle. It wasn't a trend to them but was a way of life, which they believe goes way back to the manner in which their ancestors lived for years and years. What I loved is how Yin and Yang was more than just a cool symbol. It was the balance of life and how both complemented each other. Could sleep be the integral part to balancing our lifestyle? Have you managed to completely switch off from the stress and effort of our daily lifestyle?

I really understood the meaning of quality sleep only when I experienced it, and that was rare. The ability to switch off the brain as well as the body was challenging for me as I attributed both as the same. I would go to bed at times physically exhausted but not able to sleep because my mind was still working and thinking about the next day's plan and what I needed to achieve and how I would achieve it. The solution to that was to set out my plans better, so I learned to switch off completely when it was "me" time. My wife would go to bed at times knowing I have had a long day and needed the rest, telling me I should go to bed soon, but I needed to unwind my brain before retiring for the day. We all have the same hours in the day, but we control how to get through them. So, always be mindful of your own time and how valuable it is. As we get older, we experience enough to shape how we spend our times with our loved ones, family, and work. Use the dominos in this book to be able to line them up the way you choose which benefits you most.

I wrote this book to simplify health and fitness and to cover a broad variety of topics that would assist the audience with tools that promote a habitual sustainable lifestyle. In fact, a much younger version of me would have really appreciated all these steps and would probably be in better shape both mentally and physically if I had a blueprint of the obstacles I would face. Little did I know the personal challenges I would face when I sat down to write this book. It just seemed like a great idea to write the unspoken rules of all the years of education and experience I have accumulated to create a simplified user-friendly shortcut for everyone. I bought and read several fantastic books, which helped a lot—some I finished, some I'm yet to complete but they sounded cool at the time. The more I learned, the more I wrote, and the more I wrote, the more I became reluctant to release. As the publisher forecasted, the person I am today was very different to the person who started writing this book for you to read.

The reason why I chose to use five dominos as the chapters I highlighted was because I felt a lot of people could relate to at least one of them, which would result in a chain reaction for achieving the right balance for a holistic, sustainable, healthy lifestyle. If one of the dominos was neglected or not given the attention required, the chances of one effecting the other would be high when it came to longevity. Highlighting health and fitness nuggets in this book will help raise awareness and simplify factors that would influence a family to make the right choices and enjoy the process.

One thing I have grown into and embraced a lot more that can be relevant in any industry we live, breathe, and work in is the universal law of reciprocation or laws of attraction, as some of you may have heard before. Applying this law regardless of your background, culture, religion, or social status can come a long way when practiced. It's at the center of virtually every religious, moral, and ethical system in the world, which when applied the correct way and practiced can give you back so much without your even expecting it. The problem we face in modern society is that we demand a lot without actually giving as much, whether it's time, love, energy, or hard work. The more you give wholeheartedly, in due time it comes back ten times over. It can come back and fulfill so many boxes—from self-esteem, pride, satisfaction, or even a financial benefit, to just being the best version of you. Smiling or expressing how much you appreciate someone for a simple job they do for you can come a long way and change the outcome of that person's day. It's actually contagious and free of charge!

Try setting that as a personal objective weekly to acknowledge and express two positive things to anyone who comes into your weekly routine. It could be anyone from a family member to someone you come across in the gym or serving you at a restaurant. Every week, change the person you select, leading up to at least four people a month who you have praised or whose role you have appreciated. Be sincere in your approach, and don't expect anything back, and you have already applied good energy to that environment. I know from my own experiences that nothing is more rewarding than making a difference in someone's life. I even tell my clients that what they themselves do for achieving results and accomplishing their goals is far more inspiring than I will ever be, due to the fact that there are thousands of people out there who can relate to them. Holding yourself accountable and achieving progress every day adds responsibility on your shoulders. This also empowers others to do better for themselves, as our actions are infectious.

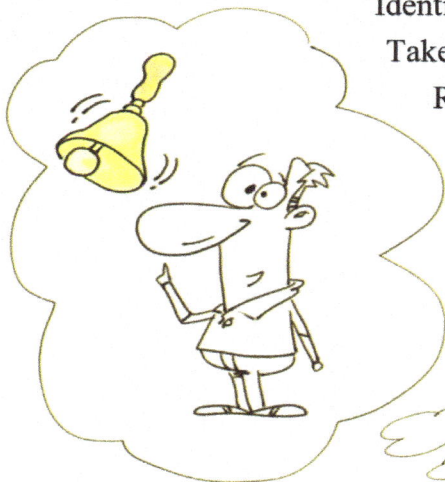

Identify Your Key Takeaways from Recovery

❖ Takeaway 1

❖ Takeaway 2

❖ Takeaway 3

❖ Takeaway 4

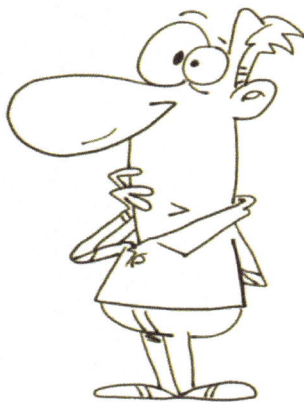

Just Gratitude

I have a lot of friends that are very poor, the only thing they have is money.

—Paul Coelho

There's always something to be grateful for, so I have attached a gratitude journal at the end of this book for you to be able to come away with more than you started.

Five Things I Am Grateful For

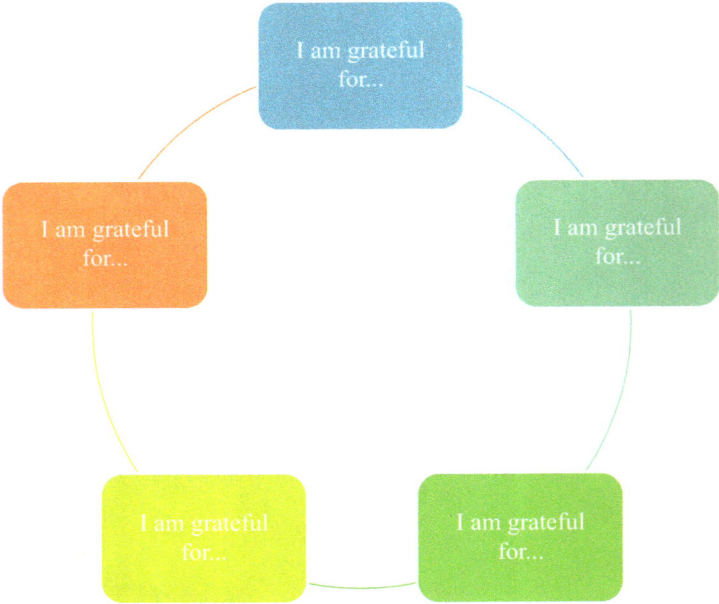

I am grateful for...

I am grateful for...

I am grateful for...

I am grateful for...

I am grateful for...

People I Am Grateful For

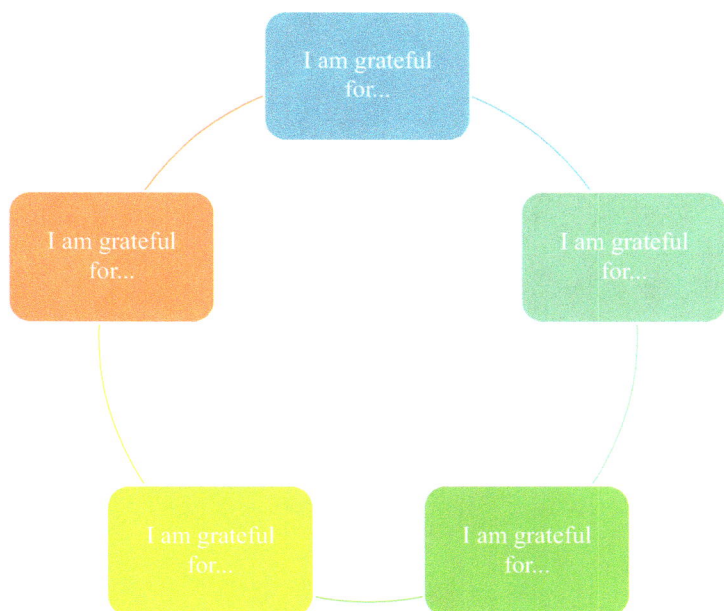

I am grateful for...

I am grateful for...

I am grateful for...

I am grateful for...

I am grateful for...

People Who Inspire Me

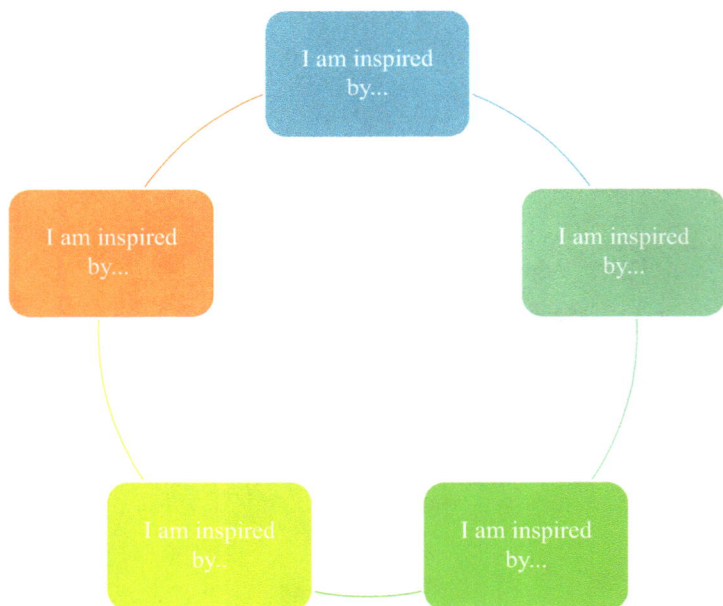

I am inspired by...

I am inspired by...

I am inspired by...

I am inspired by...

I am inspired by...

The Challenges I Am Facing

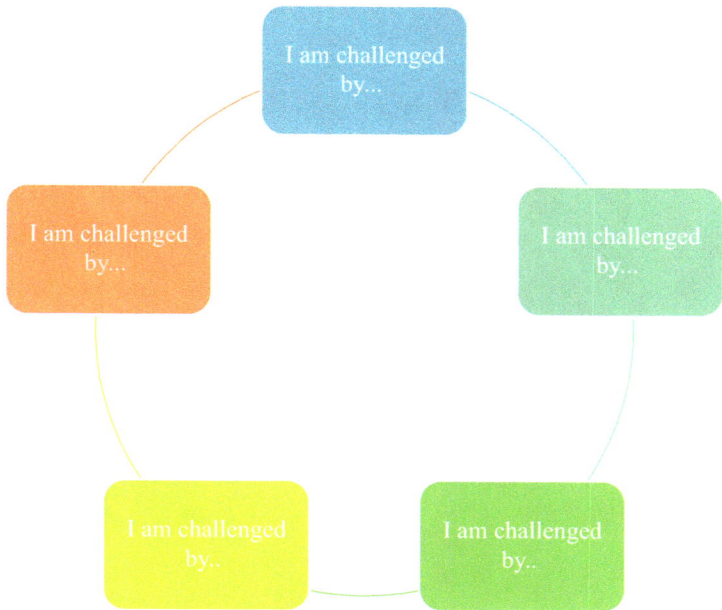

I am challenged by...

I am challenged by...

I am challenged by...

I am challenged by..

I am challenged by.

Highlight of My Day

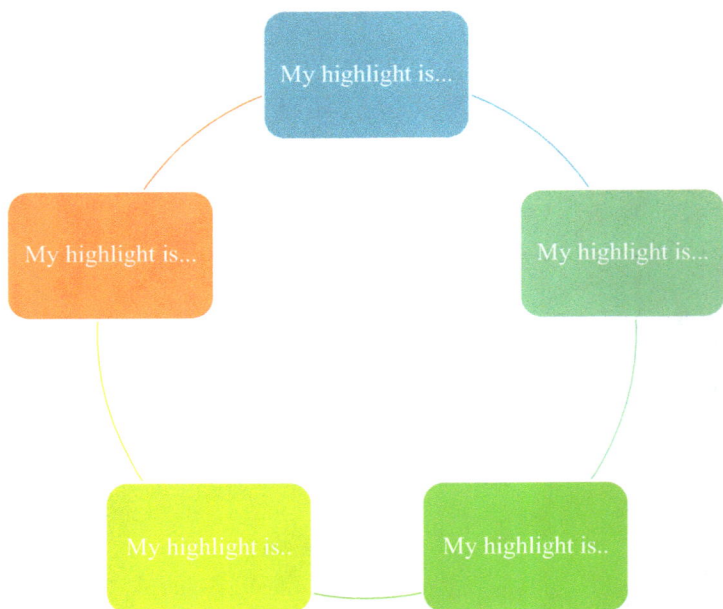

My highlight is...

My highlight is...

My highlight is...

My highlight is...

My highlight is..

Q&A's

1. Will a cheat meal really mess up my metabolism?

Because I know the person asking it on my social media, I am able to answer it directly according to his daily activities, lifestyle, and discipline in nutrition. One size definitely doesn't fit all, so before anyone out there who has already been eating freely and isn't as disciplined with nutrition and all of the above lets loose and goes "man versus food" on me, know that the answer will be different.

When sticking to a plan, a cheat meal (not day) can actually be beneficial for a number of reasons:

You appreciate the cheat meal all week, and it becomes more of a positive reward (clapping sounds from an audience).

Spiking caloric intake once per week promotes fat loss by ensuring the metabolic rate (thyroid function, etc.) resets to default even faster.

Allow five days at least of clean eating, plenty of fluids, awareness of time for meals.

Eat out for your cheat meal and devour that meal out (no leftovers brought home).

Dissecting your food at times may actually reveal what you are eating. For example, a classic cheeseburger left for a month with no visual change.

2. How important are these functions in the brain? Cerebellum? Cerebrum? Temporal lobes?

Cerebellum = It is responsible for muscle coordination, reflexes, and balance.

Cerebrum = Most of the brain function takes place in the cerebral cortex or outer layer of the cerebrum. It's the assembly line of human thought where a lot of the heavy work gets done.

Left hemisphere = The left controls your concrete side—speech, writing, language, and calculation.

Right hemisphere = The right controls your imaginative side—spatial ability.

The frontal lobes = They control things such as planning, personality, behavior, and emotion.

The parietal lobe = It is most associated with touching or moving our limbs.

Occipital lobes = They control vision.

The temporal lobes = They are located on both sides of the brain around ear level. These lobes process sound and are also responsible for short-term memory.

Brain stem = It controls the flow of messages between the brain and the body. It controls basic functions such as breathing, swallowing, consciousness, heart rate, cholesterol, and whether one is sleepy or awake.

The base or lower part of the brain is connected to the spinal cord. Together the brain and the spinal cord are known as the central nervous system (CNS). "The brain is the command center for your body, and the spinal cord is the pathway for messages sent by the brain to the body and from the body to the brain" (Learning Modules—Medical Gross Anatomy from the University of Michigan Medical School).

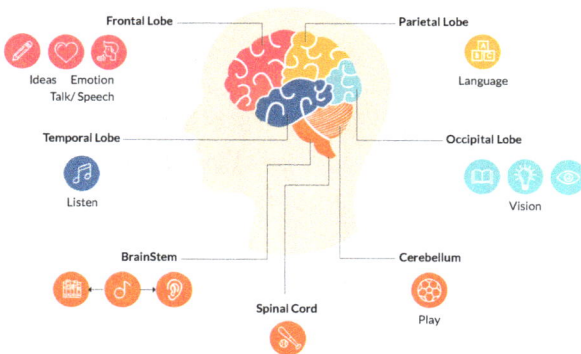

3. I see you do a lot of boxing, but would you recom-
    mend it for someone who isn't fit, or do I need to
    build my fitness up and then join?

I really don't believe you need to build up fitness to
tackle a new sport or discipline. It's actually exciting
to start something new, especially such an incredible form of exercise. The benefits are—it improves
hand-to-eye coordination, helps manage stress levels,
increases cardiovascular strength, and helps reduce
body fat while maintaining muscle mass.

Start with the basics of boxing by speaking to a coach
and listening to what they have planned, and work
your way up. It's great for both genders and a very
good workout to mix things up in your routine.

4. What is your opinion on performance versus
    aesthetics?

I think this question comes up a lot with both clients
and athletes. I tend to rephrase it slightly differently
when I assess both, especially before any physical
training is done. First, what is your objective? Is it more
about how you look? Aesthetics could be a goal they
have set in everyday life or competition nationally.
That could be a huge motive for those who want to
look better and are willing to make those sacrifices,

short and long term. My advice if you are going with that option is to allow yourself enough time to cut the weight, as your organs deserve that process. A lot has been made about how mixed martial artists lose weight for weigh-ins and dramatically cut weight and then fuel the night after. I have met some incredible specialists who focused on competing in physique shows and expressed how miserable they were despite looking fantastic on stage. With that comes a lot of deprivation and discipline from the foods they want to eat. So aesthetically they looked perfect but internally they didn't feel good at all, eventually stopping that and reverting to being healthy.

I personally feel that measuring up progress by the way you feel is a lot more sustainable and recommended for both clients and athletes. Of course, we all want to look good, but I feel you relate more to each other when you feel good and can fit into clothes that did not fit you so well a month ago—that's progress. With the dominos mentioned in this book, the aim is to be able to build that habit to make it the norm. Nutrition and training with mind-set, environment, and recovery will complete the chain. Manchester City star Sergio Aguero reset his nutrition (eliminating meat and dairy) after so many successful years in the premier league to prolong his career, becoming their all-time greatest goal scorer and won another premier league title.

5.   What are your views on intermittent fasting?

In my opinion, one of the most beneficial things I have tried when executed properly is that I followed the 16:8 rule, which was 16 hours of fasting and an 8-hour window to be able to eat your meals. However, you are allowed to hydrate with water, teas, and coffee, which help manage hydration levels, especially in a warm environment. Due to the amount of hours fasted, it also helps regulate feeling bloated or inflammatory and can reduce insulin resistance, lowering your risk of type 2 diabetes. The way our bodies work throughout the day and recover at night in most cases allows us to understand the motor reproduction of how energy is used. So, if we look at the cliché 9 to 5 in the office, our bodies will hit home at around 7 pm, after which we might be on the couch watching TV. The point is, we are less likely to be active post 8 pm, which means the link between intermittent fasting and our metabolic rate blends well and promotes weight management. The best part about intermittent fasting is that it's designed to work for you. The restrictions are only related to overcoming your mental blocks and learning to control your hunger, which will become invaluable skills once you learn that your symptoms of hunger are more because of the eating schedule you've created than actually needing food.

6. Is cortisol the enemy?

Depression and anxiety are well-known symptoms of low testosterone. Consistently high levels of cortisol, the stress hormone, can deplete the adrenal glands. There's evidence that links high levels of cortisol to the storage of abdominal fat, which explains certain cases of fat being stored around the belly. All of this makes cortisol an interesting hormone when you consider that producing it can break down fat and help you get lean, or it can cause you to store fat in the worst area when stressed. The pro is that when cortisol rises, you can use that stress to improve your performance, which is great for training. However, if cortisol remains elevated for too long, it can cause a rise in blood sugar, which makes you crave all sorts of unhealthy foods.

7. I've been advised to do weight training but despite wanting to lose weight will I get bigger and masculine?

This falls down under the classic myth that weight training makes females bulkier. In fact, a combination of weight training and cardio can double the pace at which you achieve results. Redefining your goals as getting lean is probably as close to that dream body as you will ever get. Now let's strip down that meaning by first getting an accurate assessment of what you currently weigh. I recommend Dexa Scans, calipers, or hydrostatic weighing, which involves getting dunked underwater. When analyzing your measurements, I would turn my focus to the percent of body fat, because for various reasons the BMI or overall number varies from person to person. Set a realistic goal of balancing your nutrition and training and enjoy the process. The reason I highlighted percent of body fat is because that gives you the best indication of how much of the overall weight is fat in comparison to muscle and water. I would recommend kettle-bell training, which is an incredible weight loss tool and can be utilized as weight training and cardiovascular exercise.

8. What supplements do you personally take? If you could choose just 3, what would they be?

Plant-based protein (fitness fuel) from the Hundred Wellness Clinic (Dubai, UAE), omega 3, 6, and 9 fish oils, and probiotics. The simple reason why I choose the above is because it works for me with a balanced diet to complement my training.

I hate running but hear contrasting opinions of whether it's good or not. I do lose weight from it but am worried about my knees and, quite frankly, I get bored.

My first question would be, does it hurt your knees when you run, or is that what you fear might happen? If you see results from it, then I would recommend sticking to it because it challenges you. "Repetition is the mother of skill" was said by Anthony Robbins.

Now addressing the getting bored comment, I could most definitely relate to that until I discovered the world of podcasts! The amount of information you can stimulate your brain with while you run or do something for a duration of time is wonderful and really helps from a physiological and cognitive perspective.

9. What's the number-one rule you can advise to be a successful trainer/coach?

It's hard to just have one rule, but here's my attempt to answer your question. If I could say one, it would be to develop the power of listening. Listening helps identify an issue, which makes it a lot easier to solve. Listening gives you enough time to deliver the right answer when you fully understand the client. Listen to your gut; if you feel you aren't ready, then study more, do more, and don't be afraid to take your time learning and developing. The more diverse your clientele is, the better you become at delivering the knowledge you have invested so much in. Be authentic, and don't compromise your beliefs even if the industry is swaying elsewhere, as science never changes and neither do good people.

Grateful to the support systems I have had throughout this process:

> My mum, for the unconditional love. "Paradise lies under the feet of the mother."

> My wife, for the unconditional support regardless of what frame of mind I was in throughout this process, consistently beating myself up about perfecting what I was trying to deliver.

> My friends and family, who consistently asked me when it was going to be released so they could support the cause.

> My national teams, who have enabled me to learn more by working with such incredible people from diverse backgrounds.

> Those who played vital roles in many places I visited to be in the right space to work, whether coffee shops, restaurants, or workspaces.

> My social media platforms, which interacted with me, engaged with me, and gave me the right energy and push to elevate the book.

> My publisher, Moustafa, for being on my case about delivering my story in its rawest fashion.

My coaches, who inspire me and never allow me to get ahead of myself with their brilliance, knowledge, and wisdom. Matt Coe, you have not only set the bar high in the fitness world but have continued to be the benchmark.

Maansi, for the wonderful artwork and sketches.

Dr. Sean and Ryan Penny, for their support and energy throughout this process.

Chef Victor Urbina, for looking after me and providing me with the best nutrition.

Ab for being there for me at my lowest point and searching for me all over the country.

Yassin for being Yassin.

Amr Younis, Pradeep, and Beebo, for the amazing photography.

Ahmed from Peaky blinders barbershop for always having a space on his chair whether I needed a trim or not.

London town! #mydubai & KFA

About the Author

OMAR IS AN award-winning coach, trainer, and practitioner in the health and fitness industry. A pioneer in the industry, he was educated in Europe before moving to the UAE where he has coached individuals as well as international football teams from Africa and the Middle East. He has founded his own training facility, developed a youth academy, and participated as a coach in the World Cup and African Nations Cup. His holistic approach and passion to listen, study, and help people has been recognized across the world through his long-standing relationships with athletes, clients, and celebrities.

About the Book

RESET IS A health and fitness passport on training the mind as well as the body. The five dominos are symbols of how important and vital each domino is in achieving a holistic balance when tackling life's day-to-day challenges. The book offers an insight on simplifying an overcomplicated industry. Real-life experiences and a connection with the writer are felt throughout the book, connecting the mind and the body in resetting your habits from negative to positive. From how to fuel the body to how to reset the mind before going to bed, it offers takeaways throughout the book that you can implement in your own lifestyle.

My full bio is on my website: www.omaralduri.com.
    Share your RESET journey through these hashtags on all social media platforms:
    #myresetbook
    #coachalduri

www.ingramcontent.com/pod-product-compliance
Lightning Source LLC
Chambersburg PA
CBHW062144020426
42334CB00020B/2504